Fabíola Leite da Silva

Multi-detector CT and traditional coronary angiography

Fabíola Leite da Silva

Multi-detector CT and traditional coronary angiography

Assessment of coronary artery disease

ScienciaScripts

Cover image: www.ingimage.com

This book is a translation from the original published under ISBN 978-613-9-66904-2.

Publisher:
Sciencia Scripts
is a trademark of
Dodo Books Indian Ocean Ltd. and OmniScriptum S.R.L publishing group

120 High Road, East Finchley, London, N2 9ED, United Kingdom
Str. Armeneasca 28/1, office 1, Chisinau MD-2012, Republic of Moldova, Europe
Printed at: see last page
ISBN: 978-620-8-11240-0

ACKNOWLEDGEMENTS

I would firstly like to thank **God** for giving me all the conditions and the strength to always pursue my dreams.

I would like to thank my parents **Paulo César** and **Lucimara Leite**, and my brother **Jonas Leite**, who believed in me and gave me all the support I needed to get where I am today.

I would like to thank my dear tutor Dr **Cristiane Ruiz** for her support, for believing in my ability and for the hours she gave me

I would like to thank my friends **Danielle Belo** and **Priscila Motta** for their friendship and for accompanying and supporting me on this long and difficult journey.

Finally, I would like to thank everyone who directly or indirectly contributed to the realisation of this work.

"May your efforts challenge the

remember that the great things of man have been achieved out of what seemed impossible."

Charles Chaplin

SUMMARY

CHAPTER 1	**4**
CHAPTER 2	**7**
CHAPTER 3	**11**
CHAPTER 4	**13**
CHAPTER 5	**15**
CHAPTER 6	**18**
CHAPTER 7	**20**
CHAPTER 8	**27**
CHAPTER 9	**31**
CHAPTER 10	**33**
CHAPTER 11	**34**

CHAPTER 1

INTRODUCTION

Cardiovascular diseases (CVD) prevail as the main cause of mortality in Brazil and worldwide and over the last thirty years there has been a rapid and substantial increase in developing countries, including Brazil.

According to data from the World Health Organisation (WHO), in 2012 there were 17.5 million deaths from CVD, of which 7.4 million were from coronary artery disease (CAD).

CAD is characterised by insufficient blood supply to the heart via the coronary arteries. This occurs due to a narrowing of the coronary arteries (stenosis) due to atherosclerotic plaques, thus reducing coronary blood flow and consequently reducing the supply of oxygen to the heart.

Atherosclerosis is a chronic inflammatory disease of multifactorial origin that occurs in response to endothelial aggression, mainly affecting the tunica intima of medium and large calibre arteries.

In general, the clinical manifestations of CAD, such as myocardial infarction, stroke and peripheral vascular disease, begin in middle age. However, studies indicate that the atherosclerotic process begins to develop in childhood and factors such as smoking, obesity, diabetes mellitus, hypertension, high cholesterol levels, a family history of CAD and lack of exercise increase the risk of the disease.

The standard test for diagnosing CAD is traditional/invasive coronary angiography, also called cardiac catheterisation or coronary cineangiography, which is indicated by doctors taking into account clinical aspects, the patient's gender, age and cardiovascular risk factors, as well as socioeconomic factors.

A well-done coronary angiography depends on a thorough knowledge of coronary anatomy and its variations, and on a systematic and sequential image acquisition protocol that makes it possible to visualise all coronary segments, especially areas of vessel overlap, bifurcations or tortuous anatomy. This is why it should be carried out by experienced invasive cardiologists.

For the test, left heart catheterisation is usually performed via the femoral artery, but in cases of peripheral vascular disease, access can be via the radial or brachial arteries. Catheterisation causes discomfort and requires routine monitoring and care.

Furthermore, atherosclerosis is a disease of the vessel wall, and angiography only studies its lumen, diagnosing obstructive lesions by comparing diseased segments with "supposedly" normal segments. Often, these so-called normal segments can actually exhibit the phenomenon of vessel enlargement, which occurs during the atherosclerosis process in an attempt to accommodate the plaque (positive remodelling) and only after the lumen of the vessel is compromised does this become visible on radiographic arteriography.

On examination, the percentage of coronary stenosis greater than 50% compared to the reference lumen area is considered a satisfactory criterion for indicating surgical or percutaneous intervention, depending on the location, composition and vulnerability of the atherosclerotic plaque. The description of the extent of CAD can be uniarterial, biarterial, triarterial or left main coronary lesion.

However, because it is an invasive procedure, traditional coronary angiography has the potential to leave sequelae and at least 20 per cent of diagnostic procedures using traditional coronary angiography reveal no evidence of obstructive CAD.

Another diagnostic method has been of great clinical relevance since the advent of multidetector computed tomography (MDCT) or multislice CT scanners. This has given cardiac assessment a great boost and made coronary angiography by MDCT possible.

CT was first introduced into clinical practice in 1973, with mass application beginning in the 1980s, but it wasn't until 1998 that CT scanners were introduced with the capacity for simultaneous acquisition using four rows of detectors and a minimum rotation time of 500 ms.

Since then, technological development in this area has been dizzying and there is now equipment available with 256 and even 320 rows of detectors. The progress is so great that when we look at the scans, we have the impression that we have removed a piece from inside the body, such is its materiality.

The spatial resolution of current MDCT devices is 0.4 X 0.4 X 0.4mm, which results in an isotropic voxel (with similar measurements on both sides), which is still below the spatial resolution of conventional angiography (0.1 to 0.2mm, with 8ms temporal resolution). Even so, compared to previous devices, MDCT has greater spatial and temporal resolution, managing to cover the entire volume of the heart in 8-9 s, with high clinical reliability that allows the assessment of all clinically relevant branches of the coronary tree, as well as allowing the definition of coronary stenoses.

In practice, CT can be used to assess CAD in two main ways: by determining the calcium score (CS) and by coronary angiography itself, which is based on the acquisition of a series of axial slices with submillimetre thickness covering the entire length of the heart and the images are acquired synchronously with the electrocardiogram (ECG) signal.

In order to acquire cardiovascular CT images, the patient must pause for between 10 and 15 seconds (64-detector scanner), which can vary according to the number of detectors and is within the capacity of most patients, even those with respiratory impairment.

It is also necessary to monitor the patient's electrocardiogram, which for angiotomography requires the heart rate to be as close to 60 beats per minute as possible, often requiring the use of oral or intravenous beta-blockers to achieve this rate.

Also, as with traditional coronary angiography, the test requires intravenous injection of iodinated contrast, which has potential nephrotoxic and allergenic effects, and the risk of dose-dependent reactions is related to the volume of contrast used.

CHAPTER 2

ANATOMY OF THE CORONARY ARTERIES

The heart is positioned obliquely in the thorax. The atrial and ventricular septal structures are virtually aligned, but are inclined forwards and to the left by 45 degrees in relation to a sagittal plane.

When positioned in the thorax, the heart has a sternocostal (anterior) face, which includes the right atrium, the coronary sulcus, the right ventricle, a small strip of the left ventricle and the left auricle; a diaphragmatic (inferior) face, which includes the right atrium, the coronary sulcus and both ventricles; and a base (posterior), which includes the left atrium that receives the four pulmonary veins.

The heart has four chambers: two atria, located at the top, which are the blood receiving chambers, and two ventricles, at the bottom, which are the blood ejecting chambers.

Although the heart is almost continuously filled with blood, this provides little nutrition to the cardiac tissue, as the myocardium is too thick to make diffusion a practical means of delivering nutrients, so the cardiac supply is made via the coronary circulation, which is the shortest circulation in the body.

For this, there are the heart's blood vessels, which comprise the coronary arteries and cardiac veins, which conduct the blood that enters and leaves most of the myocardium. They are integrated into the fatty tissue, cross the surface of the heart just below the epicardium and are also affected by sympathetic and parasympathetic innervation.

The right and left coronary arteries originate from the corresponding aortic sinuses in the proximal region of the ascending part of the aorta, immediately superior to the aortic valve, and run along opposite sides of the pulmonary trunk (figures 1 and 2), and their function is to supply the atria and ventricles with oxygenated blood. They circulate the heart in the coronary sulcus, with the marginal and interventricular branches in the interventricular sulcus, converging towards the apex of the heart.

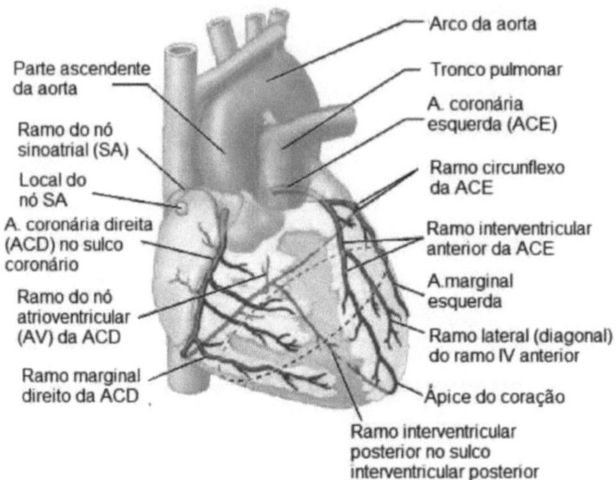

Figura 1 - Coronary arteries (anterior view)

Source: (MOORE, DALLERY, AGUR, 2014).

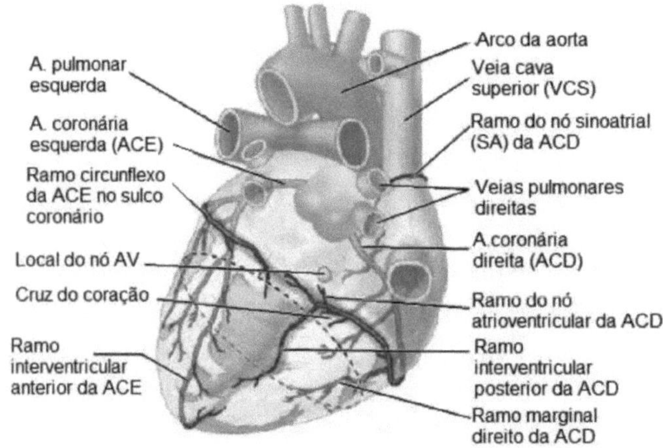

Figura 2 - Coronary arteries (posteroinferior view)

Source: (MOORE, DALLERY, AGUR, 2014).

The right coronary artery (figure 3) runs along the right side of the heart, where it divides into two branches: the right marginal branch and the posterior interventricular branch.

Near the apex of the heart, this artery fuses (anastomoses) with the anterior interventricular artery.

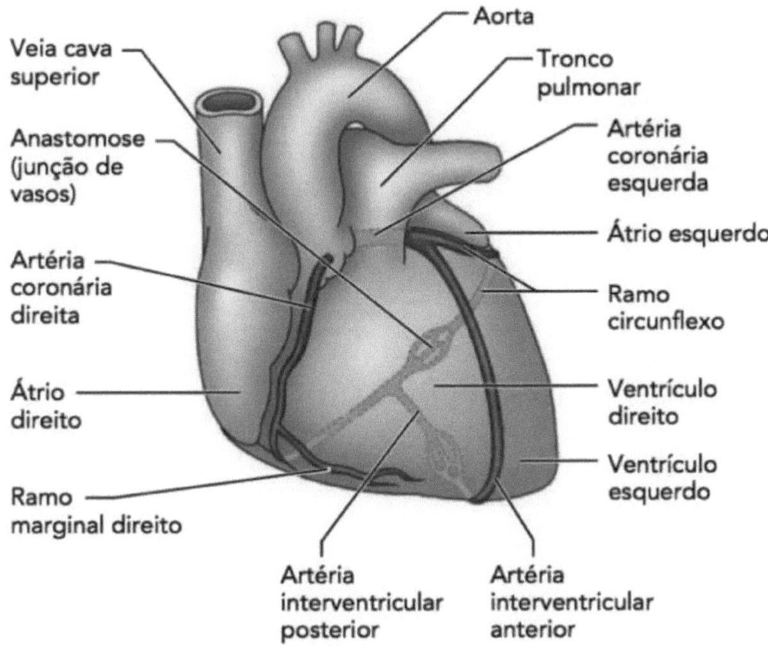

Figure 3 - Coronary circulation, main arteries (The lighter coloured vessels are located later in the heart)

Source: (MARIEB; HOEHN, 2008).

Together, the branches of the right coronary artery supply: the right atrium, the right ventricle, the sinoatrial and atrioventricular nodes, the interatrial septum, part of the left atrium, the posterior-inferior third of the interventricular septum and a portion of the posterior part of the left ventricle.

The left coronary artery runs towards the left side of the heart and divides into its main branches (figure 4): the anterior interventricular branch, which runs through the anterior interventricular groove and supplies blood to the interventricular septum and the anterior walls of both ventricles; and the circumflex branch, which supplies the left atrium and the posterior walls of the left ventricle.

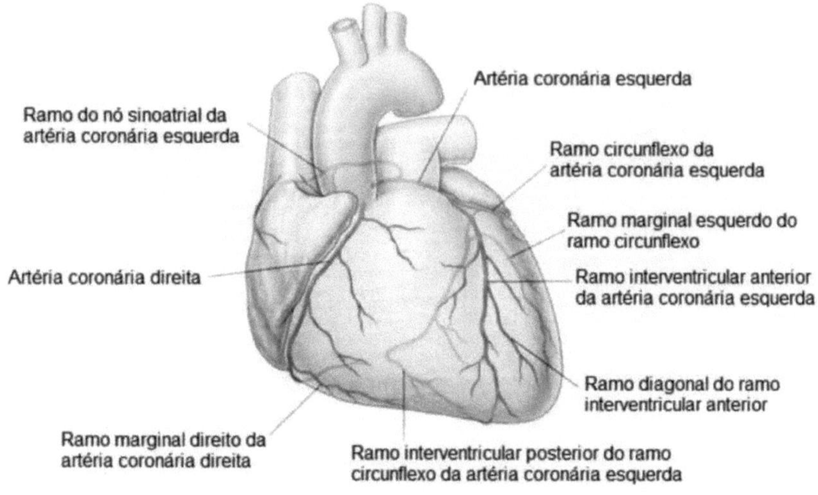

Figure 4 - Coronary arteries, main arteries and their branches

Source: (DRAKE; VOGL; MITCHELL, 2015).

CHAPTER 3

CORONARY ARTERY DISEASE

CAD is an important socio-epidemiological problem. According to the WHO, 7.4 million deaths from CAD were recorded in 2012. And to this day the disease remains the leading cause of death in developed countries.

CAD is an important manifestation of atherosclerosis and the main risk factors for developing the disease are: systemic arterial hypertension, diabetes mellitus, sedentary lifestyle, smoking, dyslipidemia, obesity and genetic factors (family history).

Atherosclerosis predominantly affects the first few centimetres of the anterior interventricular branch and the left circumflex artery, or the entire length of the right coronary artery, but in addition to affecting one of the three epicardial coronary arteries, it can also affect all of them and their branches.

Atherosclerosis is characterised by lesions in the intima called atheromas (or atheromatous or atherosclerotic plaques), where these plaques are raised lesions composed of a soft, lumpy centre of lipids (mainly cholesterol and cholesterol esters, with necrotic remains), covered by a fibrous capsule.

There are two types of atherosclerotic lesion: fixed or stable plaques, which obstruct blood flow and contribute to stable angina; and unstable or vulnerable plaques, which can rupture (spontaneously or triggered by haemodynamic factors such as blood flow or vessel tension), causing platelets to stick together and thrombus formation, which contributes to unstable angina and myocardial infarction.

In general, the clinical manifestations of CAD, such as myocardial infarction, stroke and peripheral vascular disease, begin in middle age, but atherosclerotic processes start to develop in childhood.

Atherosclerosis is produced by the following pathogenic events:

L Endothelial injury - and consequently endothelial dysfunction causing increased permeability, leukocyte adhesion and thrombosis

- Accumulation of lipoproteins (mainly oxidised LDL and cholesterol crystals in the vessel wall)
- Platelet adhesion
- Monocyte adhesion to the endothelium, migration to the intima and differentiation into macrophages and foam cells
- Accumulation of lipids inside macrophages and foam cells
- Accumulation of lipids inside macrophages, with release of inflammatory cytokines
- Recruitment of smooth muscle cells due to factors released by the activation of platelets, macrophages and vascular wall cells
- Proliferation of smooth muscle cells and production of cardiac striated muscle (CSM)

As a result of this endothelial dysfunction, harmful changes occur in vascular biology, including a decrease in the bioavailability of nitric oxide (NO), an increase in the formation of free radicals (LR) and an increase in endothelial activity. This can lead to impaired vasodilator capacity and has a direct influence on the clinical course of this and other cardiovascular diseases, such as hypertension and heart failure.

Occlusion of a large coronary artery will lead to inadequate oxygenation of an area of the myocardium and cell death, and the severity of the problem will be related to the size and location of the artery involved, whether or not the occlusion is complete, and whether or not collateral vessels are providing perfusion to the territory from other vessels.

CHAPTER 4

ANGIOGRAPHY - GENERAL ASPECTS

The angiographic study involves injecting contrast into the vascular system and visualising it using X-rays. Access can be via the femoral, radial or brachial arteries, using the Seldinger, Judkins or Sones techniques.

Before starting angiography, a medical history should be obtained, including questions to assess the patient's ability to tolerate the injection of contrast medium (e.g. allergic history, cardiac/pulmonary status and renal function), plus a medication history, because if the patient uses anticoagulants they will cause excessive bleeding during and after the procedure.

After catheterisation and the injection of contrast into the patient's vascular system, high-quality digital imaging equipment is used to acquire the images, with real-time acquisition, an essential condition for proper diagnostic judgement, as well as for optimising the outcome of the intervention.

An angiography room is larger than conventional radiography rooms and features a cleaning area with a sink and brushing equipment and a patient waiting room with oxygen and suction outlets.

The equipment is usually assembled with two X-ray tubes together with the fluoroscopic system attached to a C- or U-shaped arch, which can perform rotational and oblique movements, providing flexibility to work with postero-anterior, lateral and oblique projections.

After the angiographic procedure, patients are monitored for up to four hours and can remain hospitalised in the event of any complications.

Complications (figure 5) can be graded according to their severity and classified into nine categories: allergic, ischaemic, vascular, arrhythmic, vaso-vagal, pyogenic, neurological, embolic and congestive.

Allergic:	1.	Mild: skin manifestations
	2.	Moderate: hypotension, reversible bronchospasm
	3.	Important: previous situations that evolved into shock and/or death
Ischaemic	1.	Mild: angina controlled with nitrate
	2.	Moderate: severe angina and/or progresses to acute pulmonary oedema or low cardiac output
	3.	Important: emergency revascularisation, intra-artery or death
Vascular	1.	Mild: haematoma or minor bleeding, arterial spasm
	2.	Moderate: moderate haematoma or bleeding, need for re-intervention, arterial spasm requiring intervention
	3.	Important: large haematoma, heavy bleeding or arterial occlusion requiring surgery
Arrhythmic	1.	Mild: supraventricular tachyarrhythmia, ventricular extrasystole or sinus bradycardia
	2.	Moderate: ventricular tachycardia or fibrillation, prolonged asystole
	3.	Important: need for electrical cardioversion or pacemaker
Vagai	1.	Mild: nausea, vomiting, sweating or paleness
	2.	Moderate: bradyarrhythmia, hypotension requiring volume and/or medication
	3.	Important: previous condition that evolves into acute pulmonary oedema, myocardial infarction or asystole
Pyrogenic	1.	Mild: hyperthermia
	2.	Moderate: bacteraemia (hyperthermia, cyanosis, chills and tremors)
	3.	Important: hyperthermia with hypotension or shock
Neurological	1.	Mild: drowsiness, diplopia, dizziness
	2.	Moderate: partially reversible manifestations
	3.	Important: irreversible manifestations
Embolic	1.	Mild: peripheral embolism with no repercussions
	2.	Moderate: reversible peripheral or central embolism
	3.	Important: irreversible embolism, death
Congestive	1.	Lightweight: Killip I
	2.	Moderate: Killip II
	3.	Important: APE, cardiogenic shock

APE = Acute Pulmonary Oedema.

Figura 5 - Categorisation of complications and their severity

Source: (ROSSATO et al., 2007).

CHAPTER 5

TRADITIONAL CORONARY ANGIOGRAPHY

Over the last few decades, traditional coronary angiography has been the main imaging method for assessing coronary artery lesions, but it has significant limitations, as it allows the lumen of the vessel to be assessed, but does not evaluate its walls, providing a suggestive diagnosis.

Coronary angiography aims to define the presence of severe obstructive lesions (stenosis > 50% to 70%), the extent of the arterial involvement of the disease, i.e. the number of vessels with stenosis (classifying them as uni-, bi- or tri-arterial) and the state of the ventricle's systolic function. Knowing this information makes it possible to estimate the prognosis and define whether, in addition to treating the disease clinically, there is a need for a myocardial revascularisation procedure (angioplasty or surgery).

The degree of narrowing of the lesions is determined by visually comparing the segment of the lesion with the supposedly **"normal" distal or** proximal segment. However, in many patients, CAD is diffuse (figure 6-C) rather than focal (figure 6-A), meaning that the assessment of **"normal" reference segments is not truly normal, and that** the most pronounced lesion is underestimated.

There is also a mechanism called the "remodelling phenomenon" (figure 7) caused by the permanence of the inflammatory response and consequent weakening of the arterial wall.

Positive remodelling delays the onset of luminal loss secondary to atherosclerosis, due to the expansion of the vessel containing the plaque, and is often related to plaque vulnerability and acute ischaemic syndromes. On the other hand, negative remodelling can contribute - at the expense of vessel shrinkage - to the development of localised coronary stenosis and can be associated with stable plaque.

A study by Fattah et al. (2013) evaluating atherosclerotic plaques in vessels with positive and negative remodelling, came to the conclusion that in positive remodelling the plaques had a morphology more compatible with vulnerable plaque, of which 56% had a thin fibrotic cap, while in negative remodelling the plaques had a more stable appearance, in which 64% had pathological thickening of the intima without any evidence of fibroatheroma with a thin fibrotic cap.

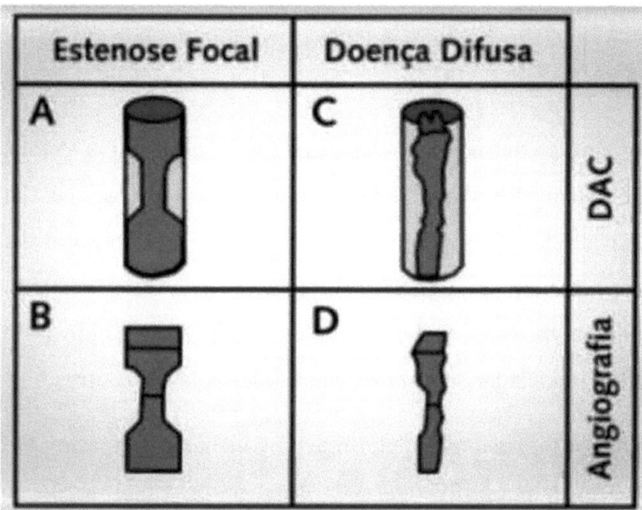

Figure 6 - Limitations of angiography in diffuse CAD. In cases C and D, angiography underestimates the severity of the stenosis.

Source: (SILVEIRA, 2002).

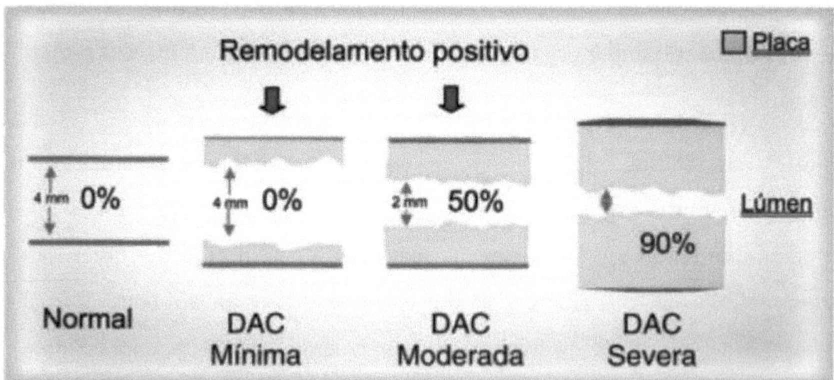

Figure 7 - Positive remodelling and stages of CAD

Source: (SILVEIRA, 2002).

As an invasive procedure, traditional coronary angiography has a 0.37% incidence of allergic reactions to the use of contrast, cardiac catheterisation has a major complication rate of 1.7%, including mortality in 0.11%, myocardial infarction in 0.05%, neurological complications in 0.07% and haemodynamic complications in 0.26% of cases.

Furthermore, at least 20% of diagnostic procedures using traditional coronary angiography reveal no evidence of obstructive CAD and approximately 40% of the patients examined have angiographically insignificant lesions.

Table 1 - Value of the traditional coronary angiography test

Hospitals/clinics	Exam Price (R$)
Albert Einstein Hospital	5.553,83
Bandeirantes Hospital	2.900,00
Oswaldo Cruz German Hospital	6.300,00
Fleury	They don't
Delboni	They don't
Nipo Brasileiro Hospital	5.393,00
Average price	**R$ 5.036,71**

A survey of the main venues that perform traditional coronary angiography in São Paulo (table 1) shows that the price of the test can reach an average of R$5,036.71, including the anaesthetist, radiologist and use of the haemodynamics room.

CHAPTER 6

COMPUTERISED TOMOGRAPHY - GENERAL ASPECTS

CT emerged as a diagnostic method in the 1970s by electronic engineer Sir Godfrey N. Hounsfield. Since its invention, the systems have evolved a few generations, where the difference between each generation is primarily related to the number and arrangement of the detectors;

The radiographic term tomography derives from the Greek word *tomos,* meaning "cuts", where anatomical sections are imaged in the axial, sagittal or coronal planes using a complex computer and a mechanical imaging system.

The basic principle of CT is based on the emission of a helix-shaped X-ray beam that passes through the body at various angles. The projection of these rays is collected by detectors at the other end of the device and this information is transformed into digital points, where each of these points is measured from a reference unit called a Hounsfield unit (HU), with the recommended value being 0 HU for water, -1000 HU for air and +1000 HU for cortical bone. Thus, based on this scale of 2000 different values, it is possible to define the density of the different tissues affected by X-rays.

According to density, images can be classified as:

- Hyperdense. High atomic number, (bone, contrast).
- Isodense. Average density scale (water and soft tissue).
- Hypodense. Low structure density (fat, air).

CT systems have three basic components - the *gantry (which* contains the X-ray tube, detector arc and collimators), the computer and the operator's console, which is used by the radiographer to operate the equipment.

The inside of the *gantry* is circular and the table with the patient is positioned at its isocentre. The entire *gantry* rotates around the patient to obtain an image or slice, knowing that the tube and detectors are positioned on opposite sides.

The X-ray tube is similar to the general radiology tube in its construction and operation. X-rays are a form of electromagnetic energy that propagates through space and is absorbed or scattered by interactions with atoms.

On the opposite side, as already mentioned, there is a series of detectors that transform the radiation into an electrical signal that is converted into a digital image.

CT uses two collimators - pre-patient (in the X-ray tube) and post-patient (in the detector) - which determine the thickness of the slice. Proper collimation reduces the dose to the patient by restricting the volume of tissue irradiated.

The digital image presentation matrix is made up of rows and columns of small blocks called picture elements. The matrices used in current equipment are 256x256, 320x320, 512x512 and 1024x1024 pixels. The number of pixels in the tomographic image represents the resolution of each point in the structure being studied and is therefore the two-dimensional representation of a corresponding volume of tissue, the voxel.

The greater the number of pixels in a matrix, the better its spatial resolution, which allows for better spatial differentiation between structures. At best, the special resolution of volumetric MDCT is 0.4 x 0.4 x 0.4 mm^3 , while the resolution of conventional radiological angiography is around 0.2 x 0.2 mm^3 .

Revolution represents a 360° rotation of the tube-detector assembly around the patient; Pitch is the ratio between the table displacement multiplied by the tube rotation divided by the slice thickness and temporal resolution determines how quickly rapidly changing signals can be recorded.

CHAPTER 7

MULTI-DETECTOR COMPUTED TOMOGRAPHY ANGIOGRAPHY

CT can be used to assess CAD in two main ways: by determining the coronary CE (figure 8), which before MDCT was done by *electron-beam computed tomography,* and by coronary angiography itself (figure 9*).*

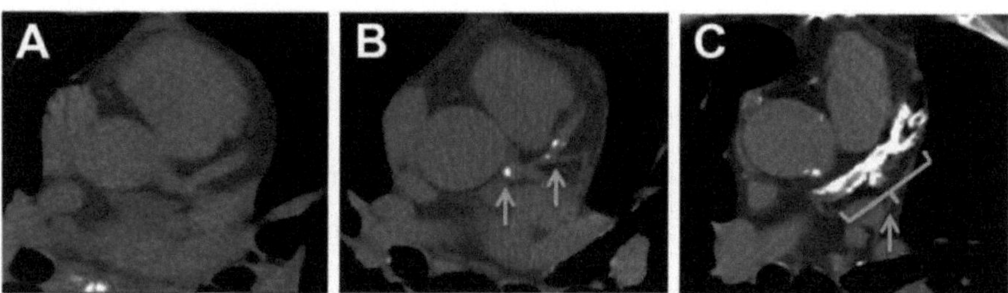

Figure 8 - Illustrative images of the coronary calcium score of three patients with increasing degrees of calcification in the anterior descending artery territory: A. no calcification; **B.** mild calcification; **C.** marked calcification.

Source: (AZEVEDO; ROCHITTE; LIMA, 2012).

CT angiography only became possible with the advent of MDCT devices in the late 1990s, and the first major attempt to outline appropriate clinical indications for cardiac CT was published by the *American College of Cardiology Foundation,* together with specialist and subspecialist societies.

It has become an important non-invasive diagnostic technique in cardiac imaging, just as traditional coronary angiography can correctly assess the extent of CAD, showing excellent accuracy in identifying or excluding the presence of significant obstructive lesions, and providing valuable prognostic information on cardiovascular risk.

Although clinical application has been possible with 16-channel devices, coronary angiography exams require the use of devices with 64 or more channels, mainly due to their greater longitudinal coverage and better spatial and temporal resolution.

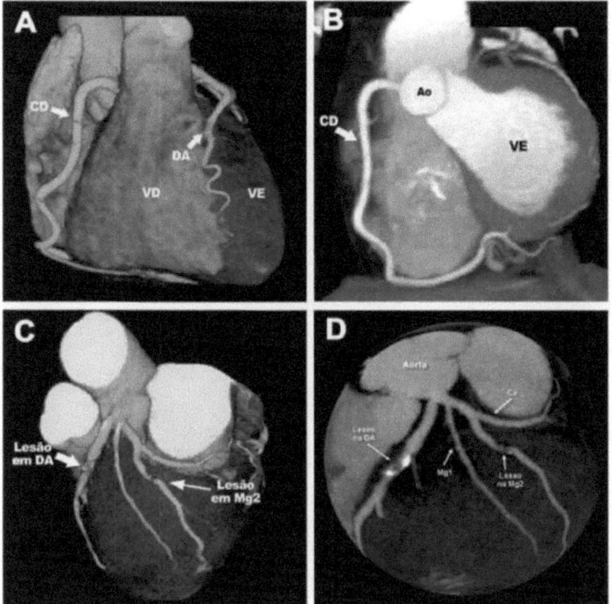

Figure 9 - Illustrative images of two patients who underwent coronary angiography. In the first patient, the angiotomography was entirely normal, excluding the presence of significant CAD (A and B). In the second patient, the scan showed two significant obstructive lesions, one at the end of the proximal third of the anterior descending artery and the other in the middle third of the second marginal branch of the circumflex artery (C and D).

Source: (AZEVEDO; ROCHITTE; LIMA, 2012).

Devices with two simultaneous X-ray sources with 64 detectors for each generator tube achieve a spatial resolution of 83 ms, very close to the **ideal** resolution of **50 ms for "freezing" the cardiac image regardless of the** number of beats per minute.

Coronary CT angiography is based on the acquisition of a series of submillimetre-thick axial slices covering the entire length of the heart and the images are synchronised to the ECG signal, which can be of the prospective sequential or retrospective helical type.

In the retrospective method (figure 10) volumetric CT data is acquired throughout the cardiac cycle during simultaneous ECG signal data. This method has the advantage of being able to order the ECG reference points for adjusting data obtained during an irregular heart rhythm, but there is the disadvantage of a higher radiation dose.

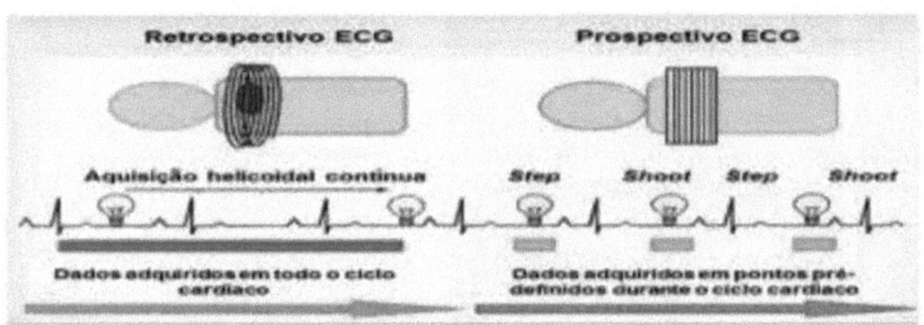

Figure 10 - ECG diagram: Retrospective and Prospective

Source: (BRAGHINI; SETTI; SCHNEIDER JUNIOR, 2014).

Unlike the retrospective method, the prospective ECG method (figure 10) allows data to be acquired by selectively rotating the X-ray tube only in the selected phase, triggered by the ECG signal and switched off for the rest of the R-R cycle, a technique also known as *step-and-shot*.

The advantage of this method is the speed of scanning and the reduction in radiation dose; however, the variation in heart rate means that data has to be acquired at different points during the cardiac cycle, resulting in artefacts, incorrect recording and low resolution.

In a study by Braghini, Setti and Schneider Junior (2014), 30 patients aged between 44 and 85, divided into two groups of 15 people each, underwent coronary angiography using 64-detector MDCT. One group underwent the exam using the prospective method and the other retrospectively to assess the difference in radiation dose.

The prospective ECG acquisition mode showed a mean effective dose of 6.8426 mSv, compared to 24.2713 mSv for the retrospective mode. The standard deviation of the observed results showed a dose increase almost six times greater in patients submitted to the retrospective method.

In another study, Gerber et al. (2009), also using a 64-detector MDCT, say that the amount of radiation from a retrospective acquisition with dose modulation is around 9.0 mSv, while the effective dose from a prospective acquisition is around 3.0 mSv.

In the scan, the images of the coronary arteries are acquired in neutral axial projection and the heart is studied in its oblique plane, because the body axis (A) is perpendicular to the CT *gantry* (C) so the cardiac axis (B) in the chest cavity is orientated obliquely (figure 11).

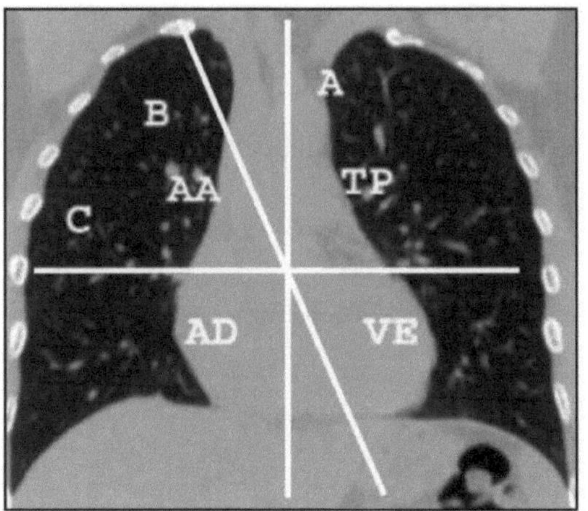

Figure 11 - Position of the heart in the thoracic cavity and axes (**AA**, ascending aorta; **PT**, pulmonary trunk; **LV**, left ventricle; **RA**, right atrium).

Source: (ANDRADE, 2006).

To better visualise the arteries, around 80-120 ml of contrast medium is used, 25% less than in traditional coronary angiography. In tomography, contrast is divided into high and low osmolality in relation to blood and also into ionic and non-ionic, where high osmolality contrasts are more likely to cause adverse reactions and are not routinely used in coronary tomography exams, and non-ionic contrasts cause fewer adverse effects, with cost being the main factor limiting their indiscriminate use.

In addition, two types of movement, respiratory and cardiac, must be controlled during CT imaging of the coronary arteries. Often a 64-detector MDCT requires an apnoea time of 10 to 15 seconds (which can be shorter with 128-detector CT or more), and these are within the capacity of most patients, even those with respiratory impairment.

Heart rate is normally controlled by beta-blockers, which slow down movement, and with a slow heart rate of between 50 and 65 beats per minute, the ECG can be used to select (retrospectively) the portion of the cardiac cycle in which coronary segment movement is at a minimum.

According to the *American College of Radiology - 2006,* this test is indicated for patients with:

- Atypical and unexplained chest pain, which could be caused by changes in the coronary artery;
- atypical and unexplained chest pain, with low or intermediate predisposition to coronary artery disease based on gender, age and risk factors;
- typical and atypical chest pain with stress test and normal or altered electrocardiographic findings;
- acute, unexplained chest pain in an acute episode with no previous clinical history of coronary artery disease. It can be used in a rapid screening to assess the presence of coronary artery disease and exclude pulmonary embolism and aortic dissection;
- coronary *by-pass* and who have new and recurrent symptoms of chest pain

In symptomatic patients with an intermediate pre-test probability of CAD, MDCT coronary angiography is the first choice of diagnostic investigation. A normal MDCT angiography and a negative calcium count can rule out invasive cardiac catheterisation in a significant percentage of patients, and pre-select patients who require an invasive procedure.

However, MDCT angiography is not recommended for patients presenting to the emergency department with acute coronary syndrome and high-risk characteristics. These patients benefit from an invasive strategy with immediate cardiac catheterisation and revascularisation. Low to intermediate risk requires additional stratification, usually necessitating the administration of these patients to hospital for exclusion or confirmation of a diagnosis.

The limitations of MDCT coronary angiography are only related to the radiation dose and the need for intravenous contrast injection, but the contrast scan has shown its potential for visualising the coronary artery wall and delineating calcified and non-calcified atherosclerotic plaques.

In the case of positive remodelling, which can underestimate the presence of CAD by traditional coronary angiography, it can be clearly visualised by a MDCT (figure 12).

The use of CT angiography as a first-line test for the assessment of chest pain in the emergency room is currently being explored, but it is already known that the test can play a role in detecting obstructive coronary disease in patients who may be inadvertently released from the emergency room.

This is because the high spatial and temporal resolution of MDCT allows both cardiac and non-cardiac causes of chest pain to be revealed and makes it possible to exclude alternative diagnoses of potentially fatal diseases, such as pulmonary embolism and aortic dissection.

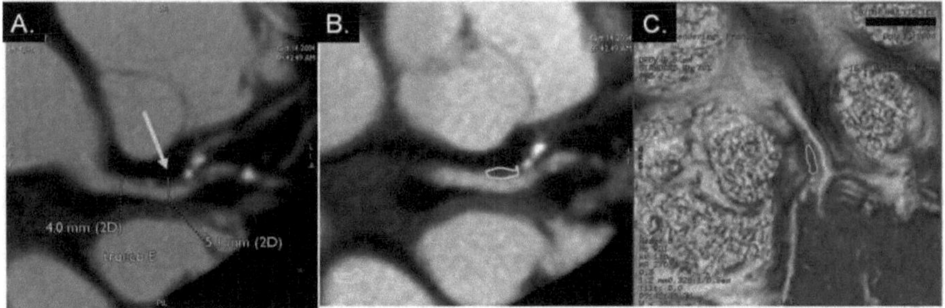

Figure 12 - Positive remodelling - CT. In A, evaluation of the left main coronary artery, identifying positive remodelling (measured in the figure), with partially calcified plaques. In B, soft plaque volume for density assessment. In C, 3D reconstruction.

Source: (HOCHHEGGER; CORDENONSI, 2013).

A survey of the main sites that perform coronary angiography by MDCT in São Paulo (table 2) shows that the price of the exam can reach an average of R$1,908.07, including the contrast medium kit.

Table 2 - Value of MDCT coronary angiography examination

Hospitals/clinics	**Exam Price (R$)**
Albert Einstein Hospital	3.017,07
Bandeirantes Hospital	980,00
Oswaldo Cruz German Hospital	1.458,00
Fleury	2.706,00
Delboni	1.420,00
Nipo Brasileiro Hospital	1.867,33
Average price	**R$ 1.908,07**

CHAPTER 8

MAIN COMPARATIVE STUDIES BETWEEN TRADITIONAL CORONARY ANGIOGRAPHY AND TCMD CORONARY ANGIOGRAPHY

Stein et al. (2008) searched PubMed up to the end of 2007 and evaluated the single-centre studies carried out using 64-channel CT scanners compared with invasive coronary angiography, arriving at an average sensitivity for identifying the presence of **significant CAD (≥50% stenosis) of 98%** and an average specificity of 88%. The average prevalence of significant CAD in these studies was 61% and the PPV 93% and NPV 96%.

In the multicentre ACCURACY study carried out in the United States, 230 patients (59.1% men, mean age 57 ± 10 years) with chest pain and no CAD, referred for invasive coronary angiography, were assessed using 64-detector CT (BUDOFF et al., 2008).

The **prevalence of significant CAD was 25% for stenoses ≥50%** and **only 14% for stenoses ≥70%. The sensitivity was 94% or 95%, depending on** the threshold chosen to define the presence of significant CAD, the specificity was 82%, the NPV was 99% for both the 50% and 70% thresholds, and the PPV was only 48% for the 70% threshold and 64% for the 50% threshold (BUDOFF et al., 2008).

In another multicentre study carried out in three Dutch university hospitals, 360 patients with an indication for invasive coronary angiography were assessed by a 64-detector MDCT, and the prevalence of significant CAD was 68%, the sensitivity and specificity were 100% and 64% respectively, the PPV was 86% and the NPV was 97% (MEIJBOOM et al., 2008).

In their study, Meijboom et al. (2008) reported that the diagnostic performance of MDCT coronary angiography in detecting significant stenosis is excellent, correctly identifying stenosis in 99% of patients with significant CAD previously diagnosed by traditional coronary angiography (figure 13).

However, in their study, Meijboom et al. (2008) reported that coronary angiography using MDCT can overestimate the severity of CAD. In their analysis, 41 patients diagnosed with insignificant CAD by traditional coronary angiography were incorrectly classified as having significant CAD by MDCT coronary angiography (figure 14).

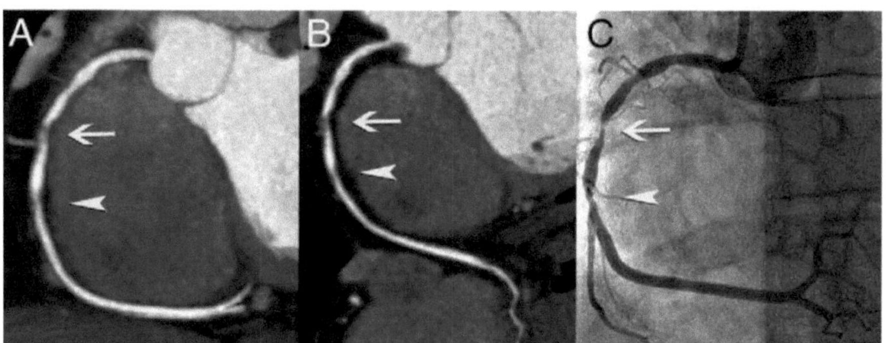

Figura 13. Right coronary artery with significant CAD. (A) Maximum intensity projected MDCT image showing the anatomy of the right coronary artery. **(B)** Multiplanar reconstruction showing a significant coronary stenosis (arrow) in the middle right coronary artery and an intermediate coronary stenosis in the distal right coronary artery (arrowhead), both corroborated by conventional coronary angiography **(C)**.

Source: (MEIJBOOM et al., 2008).

However, in their study, Meijboom et al. (2008) reported that MDCT coronary angiography can overestimate the severity of CAD. In their analysis, 41 patients diagnosed with insignificant CAD by traditional coronary angiography were incorrectly classified as having significant CAD by MDCT coronary angiography (figure 14).

Another multicentre study, known as CORE 64, in which 291 patients over the age of 40 with a clinical indication for invasive coronary angiography from 9 hospitals in 7 countries were assessed by 64-detector MDCT, the prevalence of significant CAD was 56%, sensitivity 85%, specificity 90%, PPV 91% and NPV 83% (MILLER et al., 2008).

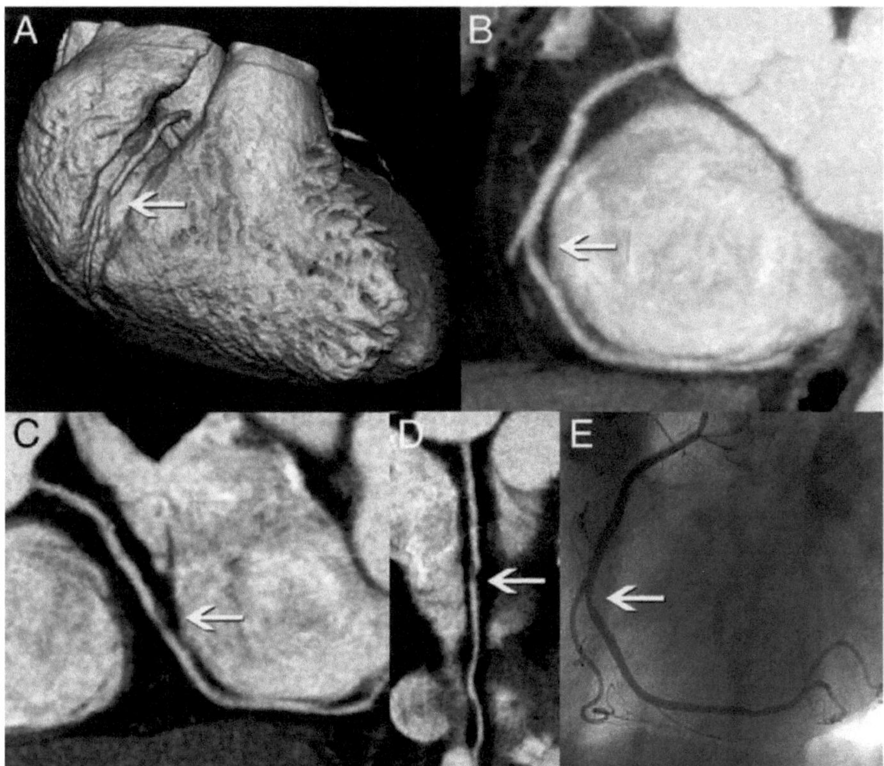

Figura 14. CAD overestimated by MDCT coronary angiography. (A) anatomy of the right coronary artery. **(B)** maximum intensity image projection. **(C, D) curved multiplanar reconstruction showing a non-calcified obstructive coronary stenosis in the right coronary artery (arrow). (E) Non-significant stenosis on conventional coronary angiography. Quantitative coronary angiography showed a 40 per cent reduction in coronary diameter.**

Source: (MEIJBOOM et al., 2008).

Comparing 64-detector CT coronary angiography with traditional coronary angiography, Fine et al. (2006) evaluated 66 patients (32 men; 62 ± 7 years old, age range 29-83 years). In total, 245 coronary arteries were assessed and in 94% of the patients an average of 50% stenosis was found, leading to a sensitivity value of 95%, specificity of 96%, PPV of 97% and NPV of 92% (FINE et al., 2006).

Schmermund (2005) also came to the conclusion that 64-detector MDCT has high diagnostic accuracy in assessing coronary artery stenoses when evaluating 67 patients (50 male and 17 female, mean age 60.1 ± 10.5 years) with suspected CAD and comparing them to invasive coronary angiography.

In his study, all **vessels ≥1.5 mm** were considered **for the** assessment of significant coronary artery stenosis (diameter reduction > 50%). 47 patients were identified as having significant coronary stenosis on invasive angiography, with 18% of the segments affected (SCHMERMUND, 2005).

The MDCT correctly identified all 20 patients with no significant stenosis on invasive angiography, achieving a sensitivity of 94%, specificity of 97%, PPV of 87% and NPV of 99% (SCHMERMUND, 2005).

Hadamitzky et al. (2011) also followed 2,223 patients with suspected CAD for a mean period of 28 months and confirmed the findings of previous studies, demonstrating that coronary angiography not only provides important prognostic information, but also that it is incremental to clinical risk scores and coronary CE.

CHAPTER 9

DISCUSSION

Conventional coronary angiography is the standard invasive test for diagnosing CAD. However, MDCT coronary angiography, especially after the introduction of the 64-channel MDCT system, has emerged as a useful technique for non-invasively ruling out CAD.

Both tests can correctly assess the extent of CAD, but MDCT coronary angiography provides a more accurate assessment of the lesion, which is usually underestimated by traditional coronary angiography, and can establish the ideal angiographic projection for eventual treatment.

This is because the assessment of CAD by traditional coronary angiography provides a two-dimensional view of a three-dimensional object, underestimates the presence of diffuse atherosclerosis and does not detect the early stages of coronary atherosclerosis.

However, MDCT can still overestimate a stenosis, classifying exams that were diagnosed as insignificant CAD by conventional coronary angiography as significant CAD.

The contrast used in both tests is the same, differing only in the volume injected. Therefore, the risk of nephrotoxic and allergenic effects applies to both tests, but the smaller the volume of contrast used in the test, the lower the risk of dose-dependent reactions.

The amount of contrast used in MDCT coronary angiography can be up to 25% less than in traditional coronary angiography. Usually, around 80 to 120ml of contrast is used in MDCT coronary angiography and around 150ml in traditional coronary angiography.

In the studies found, the authors state that MDCT can reliably rule out CAD and, furthermore, authors such as Stein et al. (2008) add that combining MDCT results with a pre-CT clinical probability assessment strengthens the diagnosis.

The high values observed in the NPVs of the authors studied, from 92% Fine et al. (2006) to 99% Schmermund (2005), with the exception of Miller et al. (2008), may establish MDCT angiography as an effective non-invasive alternative to traditional coronary angiography for ruling out obstructive coronary artery stenosis.

As has been said, the only study that argues against this diagnostic alternative is that by Miller et al. (2008), which reached a NPV of 83% and also stated that, to date, MDCT cannot replace conventional coronary angiography.

In addition, comparing the cost of both tests, we can see that the price of MDCT angiography is even more favourable than traditional coronary angiography. MDCT angiography cost an average of R$1,908.07, while traditional coronary angiography cost an average of R$5,036.71.

Traditional coronary angiography, although it is an older method than MDCT, is usually more expensive as it includes a medical team, an anaesthetist, a haemodynamics room and possible hospitalisation of the patient for post-exam evaluation.

The lowest cost found for traditional coronary angiography was at the Bandeirantes Hospital, at R$2,900.00, but this only includes 12 hours of rest, i.e. 12 hours of the patient's stay in hospital. After that, if necessary, the cost of hospitalisation and medication will be added.

In addition, some clinics such as Delboni and Fleury don't offer the service, as they don't have enough facilities to carry out such a test.

CHAPTER 10

CONCLUSIONS

The emergence of MDCT and the studies already carried out demonstrate not only that coronary angiography by MDCT has become a useful technique for detecting CAD, but also that it has the potential to replace the traditional technique.

This conclusion is directly based on the studies that have used both techniques. The vast majority of researchers are in favour of replacing traditional coronary angiography with MDCT coronary angiography for patients with suspected CAD.

The main point that makes MDCT a promising technique as a potential alternative to traditional coronary angiography is that it is preventative for patients who do not have CAD, as well as being a non-invasive method compared to traditional coronary angiography (catheterisation).

The financial factor, together with the reduction in nephrotoxic risk due to the use of contrast, also corroborates the fact that MDCT is considered an excellent test.

In terms of the structures visualised, MDCT provides a view not only of the arterial walls but also of the vessel lumen, which is not achieved in traditional coronary angiography, and therefore has greater specificity than traditional coronary angiography.

CHAPTER 11

REFERENCES

ALBUQUERQUE, Luciano C.; PALMA, José H.; BRAILE, Domingo. Guidelines for aortic disease surgery. **Arch Bras. Cardiol,** v. 82, p.35-50, mar. 2004.

ANDRADE, Joalbo Matos. Coronary anatomy with multicut computed tomography angiography. **Radiologia Brasileira,** Brasília, v. 39, n. 3, p. 233-236, jun. 2006.

AZEVEDO, Clerio F.; ROCHITTE, Carlos E.; LIMA, João A.c.. Calcium score and coronary angiography in cardiovascular risk stratification. **Arq. Bras. Cardiol.,** São Paulo, v. 98, n. 6, p. 559-568, jun. 2012.

BERTINI, Paulo J. **Non-invasive detection of atherosclerotic plaque and remodelling of coronary arteries by magnetic resonance imaging.** 2003. 82 f. Thesis (Doctorate in Cardiology) - Cardiology Course, University of São Paulo School of Medicine, São Paulo, 2003.

BONTRAGER, Kenneth L.; LAMPIGNANO, John P.. **Treatise on radiographic positioning and associated anatomy.** 6. ed. Rio de Janeiro: Elsevier, 2005. 850 p.

BRAGHINI, André L.; SETTI, João A. P.; SCHNEIDER JUNIOR, Bertoldo. Radiation dose assessment: coronary angiotomography - retrospective and prospective methods. In: XXIV Brazilian Congress of Biomedical Engineering - CBEB 2014. Rio de Janeiro. p. 1738 - 1741.

BRATS, Year III N°4: **MULTI-DETECTOR COMPUTED TOMOGRAPHY IN THE DIAGNOSIS OF ARTERIAL DISEASE CORONARY HEART DISEASE.** 2008. Available at: <http://www.ans.gov.br/images/stories/Materiais_para_pesquisa/Perfil_setor/Brats/2008_mes06_brats_04.pdf>. Accessed on: 13 Feb. 2017.

BRAUNWALD, Eugene et al. ACC/AHA 2002 guideline update for the management of patients with unstable angina and non-ST-segment elevation myocardial infarction- -summary article: a report of the American College of Cardiology/American Heart Association task force on practice guidelines (Committee on the Management of Patients With Unstable Angina). **Journal Of The American College Of Cardiology,** v. 40, n. 7, p.1366-1374, 02 Oct. 2002.

BUDOFF, Matthew J. et al. Diagnostic performance of 64-multidetector row coronary computed tomographic angiography for evaluation of coronary artery stenosis in individuals without known coronary artery disease: results from the prospective

multicentre ACCURACY (Assessment by Coronary Computed Tomographic Angiography of Individuals Undergoing Invasive Coronary Angiography) trial. **Journal Of The American College Of Cardiology,** v. 52, n. 21, p.1724-1732, 18 nov. 2008.

BUSHONG, Stewart C. **Radiological science for technologists:** physics, biology and protection. 9. ed. Rio de Janeiro: Elsevier, 2010. Translation by Sandro Martins Dolghi et. al.

CAIXETA, Adriano M. et al. Multislice Coronary Tomography with 16 Detector Columns in the Diagnosis of Arterial Remodelling. **Rev Bras Cardiol Invas,** v. 12, n. 2, p.102-103, jun. 2004.

CANEVARO, Lucía. **Interventional radiology.** Available at: <http://rle.dainf.ct.utfpr.edu.br/hipermidia/images/documentos/Radiologia_intervenci o nista.pdf>. Accessed on: 28 Feb. 2007.

CÉSAR, Luiz Antonio Machado. Stable angina chronic coronary disease guidelines. **Arq. Bras. Cardiol.,** São Paulo, v. 83, n. 2, p.1-43, 1 Sep. 2004.

CHEN, Grace; REDBERG, Rita F. Noninvasive diagnostic testing of coronary artery disease in women. **Cardiol Rev**, v. 8 n.6, p. 354-360, 2000.

CHEQUER, Graziela et al. Carotid Intima-Media Thickening and Endothelial Function in Coronary Artery Disease. **Arch Bras. Cardiol.,** Belo Horizonte, v. 87, n. 2, p.84-90, aug. 2006.

COSTA, Ricardo A.; LANSKY, Alexandra J.; REIBER, Johan H. C.. Quantitative coronary angiography: methods and applications. In: SOUSA, Amanda G.r.m. et al. **Cardiovascular Interventions**: Solaci. Bogotá: Distribuna Editorial, 2009. Chap. 19. p. 169-183.

COSTA, Denis H. (Org.) **Radiology:** basic physics, pharmacological bases applied to imaging, film processing, radiological equipment and accessories, radiological techniques, radiological anatomy and computed tomography. São Paulo: Martinari, 2009. 656 p.

DRAKE, Richard L.; VOGL, A. Wayne; MITCHELL, Adam W. M.. **Gray's clinical anatomy for students.** 3. ed. Rio de Janeiro: Elsevier, 2015. 1161 p.

FAIZ, Omar; BLACKBURN, Simon; MOFFAT, David. **Basic anatomy: an** illustrated guide to fundamental concepts. 3. ed. Barueri, Sp: Manole, 2013. Translation by Paulo Laino Cândido.

FATTAH, Tammuz et al. Association between vascular remodelling and necrotic core in coronary arteries: analysis by intracoronary ultrasound with Virtual Histology. **Revista Brasileira de Cardiologia Invasiva,** v. 21, n. 1, p.60-66, mar. 2013.

FINE, Jeffrey J. et al. Comparison of accuracy of 64-slice cardiovascular computed tomography with coronary angiography in patients with suspected coronary artery disease. **Am J Cardiol,** v. 97, n. 2, p.173-174, 25 Jan. 2006.

GALVÃO, Paulo B. de A. Technology and medicine: medical images and the doctor-patient relationship. **Revista Bioética,** v. 8, n. 1, p.127-136, 2000.

GERBER, T. C. et al. Ionizing Radiation in Cardiac Imaging: A Science Advisory From the American Heart Association Committee on Cardiac Imaging of the Council on Clinical Cardiology and Committee on Cardiovascular Imaging and Intervention of the Council on Cardiovascular Radiology and Intervention. **Circulation,** v. 119, n. 7, p.1056-1065, 9 Feb. 2009.

GHOSTINE, Said et al. Non-invasive diagnosis of ischaemic heart failure using 64-slice computed tomography. **European Heart Journal,** v. 29, n. 17, p. 2133-2140, jul. 2008.

GONZÁLEZ, Aloha Meave et al. Multidetector computed tomography of coronary arteries: state of the art. Part II: Clinical applications. **Archivos de Cardiología de México,** v. 78, n. 2, p.195-209, Apr./Jun. 2008.

GUARDADO, Jorge Humberto et al. Revascularisation of the proximal anterior descending artery with drug-coated stents. **Arch Bras. Cardiol.,** São Paulo, v. 88, n. 2, p.159-166, feb. 2007.

GUIMARÃES, Hélio Penna; AVEZUM, Álvaro; PIEGAS, Leopoldo S.. Epidemiology of acute myocardial infarction. **Revista da Sociedade de Cardiologia do Estado de São Paulo**, v. 16, n. 1, p.1-7, jan. feb. mar. 2006.

GUIMARÃES, Jorge I. (Org.) Guideline on indications for intracoronary ultrasound in clinical practice. **Arq. Bras. Cardiol.**,São Paulo, v. 81, p.1-10, 2003.

GUS, Iseu et al. Variations in the prevalence of risk factors for coronary artery disease in Rio Grande do Sul: A comparative analysis between 2002-2014. **Arq. Bras. Cardiol.**, p.573-579, 2015.

HADAMITZKY, Martin. et al. Prognostic Value of Coronary Computed Tomographic Angiography in Comparison With Calcium Scoring and Clinical Risk Scores. **Circulation: Cardiovascular Imaging**, v. 4, n. 1, p.16-23, 30 Sep. 2011.

HOCHHEGGER, Bruno; CORDENONSI, Isadora C. O. O. Cardiac computed tomography: what we should know. **Revista da Amrigs**, Porto Alegre, v. 57, n. 2, p.149-154, jun. 2013.

IBANEZ, B.; VILAHUR, G.; BADIMON, JJ.. Plaque progression and regression in atherothrombosis. **Journal Of Thrombosis And Haemostasis**, New York, p. 292299. 2007.

JACOBS, Jill E. et al. ACR Practice Guideline for the Performance and Interpretation of Cardiac Computed Tomography (CT). **Journal Of The American College Of Radiology**, v. 3, n. 9, p. 677-685, sep. 2006.

JUCHEM, Beatriz C.; **DALL' AGNOL**, Clarice M.; MAGALHÃES, Ana M. M. Iodinated contrast in computed tomography: prevention of adverse reactions. **Rev Bras Enferm**, Brasília, v. 57, n. 1, p. 56-61, 2004.

JÚNIOR, Edson; YAMASHITA, Helio. Basic aspects of computerised tomography and magnetic resonance imaging. **Brazilian Journal of Psychiatry**, v. 23, p.2-3, May 2001.

KOPP, Andreas F. et al. Non-invasive characterisation of coronary lesion morphology and composition by multislice CT: first results in comparison with intracoronary ultrasound. **European Radiology**, v. 11, n. 9, p.1607-1611, 2001.

KUMAR, Vinay; ABBAS, Abul K.; ASTER, Jon C. **Basic pathology.** 9. ed. Rio de Janeiro: Elsevier, 2013. 928 p.

LEE, Joseph K.T. et al. **Computed tomography of the body in correlation with magnetic resonance imaging.** 4. ed. Rio de Janeiro: Guanabara Koogan, 2008.

LIMA, Valter C.. Cardiac catheterisation, diagnosis (angiography) and therapy (angioplasty) in coronary artery disease in diabetic patients. **Arquivos Brasileiros de Endocrinologia & Metabologia**, v. 51, n. 2, p. 299-304, Mar. 2007.

LOSCALZO, Joseph. **Harrison's Cardiovascular Medicine**. 2. ed. São Paulo: Artmed, 2014. 499 p.

MARIEB, Elaine N.; HOEHN, Katja. **Anatomy and physiology.** 3. ed. Porto Alegre: Artmed, 2008. 1072 p.

MARK, Daniel B. et al. ACCF/ACR/AHA/NASCI/SAIP/SCAI/SCCT 2010 Expert Consensus Document on Coronary Computed Tomographic Angiography. **Journal Of The American College Of Cardiology**, v. 55, n. 23, p. 2663-2699, jun. 2010.

MATSUMOTO, Naoya et al. Non-Invasive Assessment and Clinical Strategy of Stable Coronary Artery Disease by Magnetic Resonance Imaging, Multislice Computed Tomography and Myocardial Perfusion SPECT. **Circulation Journal.** p. 34-40. Jan. 2010.

MEIJBOOM, W. Bob et al. Diagnostic Accuracy of 64-Slice Computed Tomography Coronary Angiography. **Journal Of The American College Of Cardiology,** v. 52, n. 25, p. 2135-2144, dec. 2008.

MET, Rosemarie et al. Diagnostic performance of computed tomography angiography in peripheral arterial disease: a systematic review and meta-analysis. **Jama,** v. 4, n. 301, p. 415-424, 28 Jan. 2009.

MILLER, Julie M. et al. Diagnostic Performance of Coronary Angiography by 64-Row CT. **New England Journal Of Medicine,** v. 359, n. 22, p. 2324-2336, 27 nov. 2008.

MOORE, Keith L.; DALLERY, Arthur F.; AGUR, Anne M. R.. **Clinically Oriented Anatomy.** 7. ed. Rio de Janeiro: Guanabara Koogan, 2014. 1114 p. Translation by

Claudia Lucia Caetano de Araujo.

MOWATT, Graham. et al. 64-Slice computed tomography angiography in the diagnosis and assessment of coronary artery disease: systematic review and meta-analysis. **Heart**, v. 94, n. 11, p.1386-1393, 31 jul. 2008.

MUSTELIER, Juan V. et al. Echocardiographic parameters of epicardial fat deposition and their relationship with coronary artery disease. **Arq. Bras. Cardiol.**, São Paulo, v. 97, n. 2, p.122-129, Aug. 2011.

NASCIMENTO, Jedson S. et al. Clonidine in coronary cineangiography: sedative effects on blood pressure and heart rate. **Arq. Bras. Cardiol.**, v. 87, n. 5, p. 603-608, nov. 2006.

NIEMAN, Koen et al. Coronary angiography with multi-slice computed tomography. **The Lancet**, v. 357, n. 9256, p. 599-603, feb. 2001.

ONCEL, Dilek et al. Detection of significant coronary artery stenosis with 64-section MDCT angiography. **European Journal Of Radiology**, v. 62, n. 3, p.394-405, jun. 2007.

PANNU, Harpreet K. et al. Current Concepts in Multi-Detector Row CT Evaluation of the Coronary Arteries: Principles, Techniques, and Anatomy1. **Radiographics**, v. 23, n. 1, p.111-125, oct. 2003.

PINHO, Ricardo A. et al. Coronary artery disease, physical exercise and oxidative stress. **Arq. Bras. Cardiol.**, São Paulo, v. 94, n. 4, p.549-555, Apr. 2010.

PORTH, Carol Mattson; KUNERT, Mary Pat. **Physiopathology.** 6. ed. Rio de Janeiro: Guanabara Koogan, 2004. 1450 p.

ROBERTS, W T; BAX, J J; DAVIES, L C. Cardiac CT and CT coronary angiography: technology and application. **Heart**, v. 94, n. 6, p. 781-792, 1 Jun. 2008.

ROCHA, Myrna S.; ASSUMPÇÃO, Lia R.; ARAÚJO, Denizar V. Accuracy of Multiple Detector Computed Tomography in the Diagnosis of Coronary Artery Disease: a systematic review. **Revista Brasileira de Cardiologia,** Rio de Janeiro, v. 25, n. 2, p.141-148, mar. 2012. Available at: <http://www.rbconline.org.br/wp-content/uploads/v25n02a08.pdf>. Accessed on: 14 Dec. 2015.

ROCHITTE, Carlos E. I Diretriz de Ressonância e Tomografia Cardiovascular da Sociedade Brasileira de Cardiologia: Sumário Executivo. **Arq. Bras. Cardiol.**, São Paulo, v. 87, n. 3, p. 48-59, sep. 2006.

RODRIGUES, André R. V. et al. Minimally invasive coronary angiography using multiple detector tomography. **Arq. Bras. Cardiol.**, São Paulo, v. 86, n. 5, p.323-330, May 2006.

RODRIGUEZ-GRANILLO, Gaston A.; CAMPISI, Roxana; CARRASCOSA, Patricia. Noninvasive Cardiac Imaging in Patients with Known and Suspected Coronary Artery Disease: What is in it for the Interventional Cardiologist? **Current Cardiology Reports,** New York, v. 18, n. 1, p.1-11, Jan. 2016.

ROMALDINI, Ceres C. et al. Risk factors for atherosclerosis in children and adolescents with a family history of premature coronary artery disease. **J. Pediatr. (rio J.),** Porto Alegre, v. 80, n. 2, p.135-140, Apr. 2004.

ROSSATO, Géderson et al. Analysis of hospital complications related to cardiac catheterisation. **Revista Brasileira de Cardiologia Invasiva,** v. 15, n. 1, p.44- 51, mar. 2007.

RUSSO, Vincenzo et al. Clinical value of multidetector CT coronary angiography as a preoperative screening test before non-coronary cardiac surgery. **Heart,** v. 93, n. 12, p.1591-1598, 2007.

SAAD, Jamil A.; GARCIA, José C. de F.; GUIMARÃES, Jorge I. Guidelines for diagnostic and therapeutic tests in haemodynamics. **Arq. Bras. Cardiol.,** v. 82, p.1-6, 2004.

SCHMERMUND, Axel. Non-invasive computed tomographic coronary angiography: the end of the beginning. **European Heart Journal,** v. 26, n. 15, p.1451-1453, 25 May 2005.

SCHOEPF, U. Joseph et al. Coronary CT Angiography. **Radiology,** v. 244, n. 1, p.48-63, jul. 2007.

SERRA, Daniel et al. Prognostic value of computed tomography angiography in the evaluation of coronary artery disease. **Rev de Ciências da Saúde da ESSCVP.** v. 1, p. 42-52, 2009.

SILVEIRA, Carlos A. da M. Intracoronary Ultrasound: Correlation with Angiography and Clinical Application. **Revista Brasileira de Ecocardiografia,** n. 3, p.44-53, Oct/Nov/Dec 2002.

SPOSITO, Andrei C. IV Diretriz Brasileira sobre Dislipidemias e Prevenção da Aterosclerose: Departamento de Aterosclerose da Sociedade Brasileira de Cardiologia. **Arq. Bras. Cardiol.,** São Paulo, v. 88, p.2-19, Apr. 2007.

STANDRING, Susan. **Gray's Anatomy:** The Anatomical Basis of Clinical Practice. 40. ed. Rio de Janeiro: Elsevier, 2010. 1584 p. Translation by Denise Costa Rodrigues et al.

STEIN, Paul D. et al. 64-Slice CT for Diagnosis of Coronary Artery Disease: A Systematic Review. **The American Journal Of Medicine,** v. 121, n. 8, p.715-725, aug. 2008.

SUN, Zhonghua. Multislice CT angiography in cardiac imaging: prospective ECG-gating or retrospective ECG-gating? **Biomedical Imaging And Intervention Journal,** v. 6, n. 1, p.1-7, jan. 2010.

VILES-GONZALEZ, Juan F. In Vivo 16-Slice, Multidetector-Row Computed Tomography for the Assessment of Experimental Atherosclerosis: Comparison With Magnetic Resonance Imaging and Histopathology. **Circulation,** v. 110, n. 11, p.1467-1472, 14 Sep. 2004.

VOGL, Thomas J. et al. Techniques for the Detection of Coronary Atherosclerosis: Multi-detector Row CT Coronary Angiographyl. **Radiology,** v. 223, n. 1, p.212-220, Apr. 2002.

WORLD HEALTH ORGANISATION (OMS). Cardiovascular diseases. Jan. 2015. Available at: <http://www.who.int/mediacentre/factsheets/fs317/en/>. Accessed on: 14 Jan. 2016

ZANZONICO, Pat; ROTHENBERG, Lawrence N.; STRAUSS, H. William. Radiation Exposure of Computed Tomography and Direct Intracoronary Angiography. **Journal of The American College Of Cardiology,** v. 47, n. 9, p.1846-1849, May 2006.

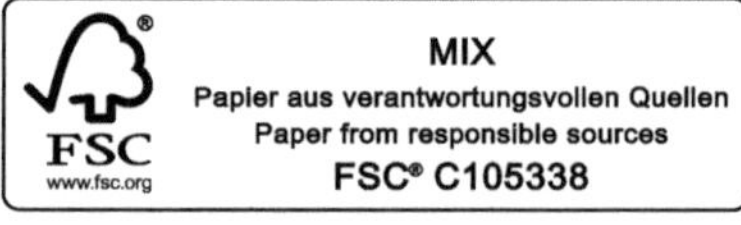

Printed by Books on Demand GmbH, Norderstedt / Germany